The Compact Book of
Being Beautiful

Jane Cunningham

summersdale

THE COMPACT BOOK OF BEING BEAUTIFUL
Copyright © Jane Cunningham, 2004
Images © Getty Images

The right of Jane Cunningham to be identified as the author of this work has been asserted in accordance with sections 77 and 78 of the Copyright, Designs and Patents Act 1988.

No part of this book may be reproduced by any means, nor transmitted, nor translated into a machine language, without the written permission of the publisher.

Summersdale Publishers Ltd
46 West Street
Chichester
West Sussex
PO19 1RP
UK

www.summersdale.com

Printed and bound by Proost, Belgium.

ISBN: 1 84024 430 5

Contents

Let's Face It...

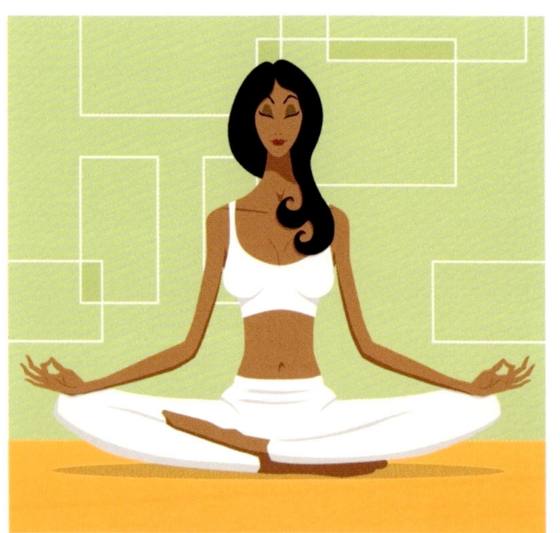

Make-up can be a minefield. Even the starriest celebrities, left to their own devices, can end up looking like a paint-factory accident. The difference between them and us, of course, is the magic fairy of make-up – the Make-Up Artist. Most celebrities won't go to the opening of an envelope without their personal pretty-painter on hand to smooth away the excesses of last night's whatever launch. But, almost without exception, everyone looks and feels that bit brighter, better and more beautiful with a helping hand from cosmetics, which is why getting your mini-manicured hands on some tricks of the trade will transform your looks from need-to-know to in-the-know. Starting right from the very beginning, settle down to step by step, straight-talking, wrinkle-smoothing, myth-busting, eye-widening, lip-plumping make-up secrets.

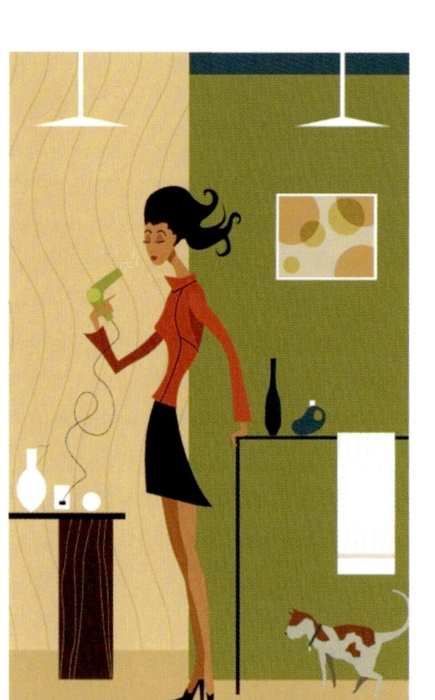

Essential Kit to Wow the World

If your make-up bag is a mish-mash of half-used eye pencils and a few squashed lippies, it's time to take stock of what is really going on in there, apart from germ warfare. The first thing you need to know is that when you are poking your eyes with brushes, pencils, fingers and anything else, you will provide party time for bacteria. Keep everything clean.

Without the essential items, there is nothing to build on, and a random selection of impulse buys does not usually make a pretty face. Your list of basics should include all of the items listed, but that doesn't mean you can't go crazy and snap up that glitter-shot, rollerball gloss if you feel like it. If you want it, you go girl!

Firstly, think of the 'essentials' as your box of crayons: without the blue, you can't do sky, right? Okay, secondly, don't panic! The list looks long, but build it up over a period of time and remember that pricey doesn't always pay. There are now so many different products available that beauty on a budget is easy-peasy. A must-have, such as foundation, is worth splashing out on, so trash the take-away for a couple of oven-readies and splash out on your face instead.

Ouch! That Hurt my Wallet…

FOUNDATION: A brilliant base is worth its weight in glittering gold because it's the start of everything you do next. Chat up the make-up dragons at the beauty counters; ask for colour advice and samples and don't be sweet-talked into buying the first one you try because the lady is nice. It's her job. You need to know how it reacts on your skin, how it looks in the cold light of day not the strip lights of the department store and most importantly you need to like the smell. This stuff is going to hang around on your face all day – if you hate the smell, tint becomes torture.

TOOLS OF THE TRADE: A really good set of brushes is a worthwhile, but pricey, investment. Go for the best you can afford and ensure that it includes big, soft brushes for blush, loose powder and shimmer; a very fine brush for lining the eyelids, both above and under; a flat brush for applying eye colour; and an eyebrow comb. Lip brushes aren't essential.

MASCARA: Great mascara doesn't flake from your eyes as the day wears on. Great mascara doesn't clump, lump and cake. Cheap ones usually do.

You Won't Need to Sell the Cat to Buy…

CREAM BLUSH: A cream blush is a cream blush is a cream blush. It's technique, not cash, that makes your cheeks glow.

LIPSTICK AND LIP GLOSS: Because of the huge trial-and-error factor in lipsticks, don't bust the bank for one. That lively, disco fandango mauve looks fabulous in the shop. You step outside and someone tries to resuscitate you…

GLOW LOTION: What? Glow lotion makes the difference between luminous skin and lacklustre skin, so look out for any face products that contain the words 'light reflective'.

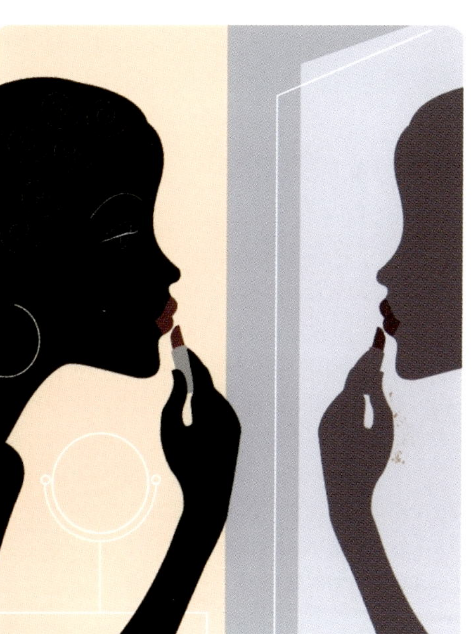

Eyelash Curlers: Since the advent of 'curling' mascaras that hold your lashes in place, these are no longer wide-eyed essentials.

Eyeliner: Just make sure the crayon is creamy soft because skin around the eye area is oh so delicate.

Eye Shadow: Check out department store own brands rather than specialised beauty counters. Many have their own range of colours and palettes made for them by the same gang who make the nicey-but-pricey stuff. Look out for a basic set of four shades, in keeping with your eye colour. For example, if you have brown eyes, a set of four shadows in the brown spectrum will see you from daytime through evening with the right application.

Cheap as Chocolate
and Better for Your Bottom…

A TUB OF VASELINE: A multi-talented, eyebrow-smoothing, lip-glossing, sheen-giving-tastic invention.

COTTON BUDS: Your mistake erasers!

Forget About…

Shimmery, glittery, sparkly stuff: As you are unlikely to want to shine your way into the office on a wet Monday morning, anything with the word 'shimmer' or similar needs to be treated carefully. Don't splash out on expensive, glittery products that are only likely to see daylight at Christmas, but do use them to vamp up an evening look.

Powder: Because it's just so OVER. Glow is good, matt is ageing. Puff powder all over your cheeks and watch them turn into a map of The Grand Canyon. Powder has a knack of clinging to crinklies. You will only ever need powder if your skin is excessively oily, you want to wear matt lipstick, or you are going to a fancy-dress ball as Queen Elizabeth I.

Nail Varnish: Think about it – do you know anyone with an empty nail varnish bottle? Have fun, experiment and consign to the file marked 'bin' when you realise you'll never wear it again.

Make-Up Artist Secret:

No eyebrow brush?

Use an old toothbrush instead.

Face Fact:

Egyptian women wore lead sulphide on their eyes to deter flies.

Good circulation is the key to good skin.
Time spent in the gym will increase your
blood flow and the results will show on
your face and body.

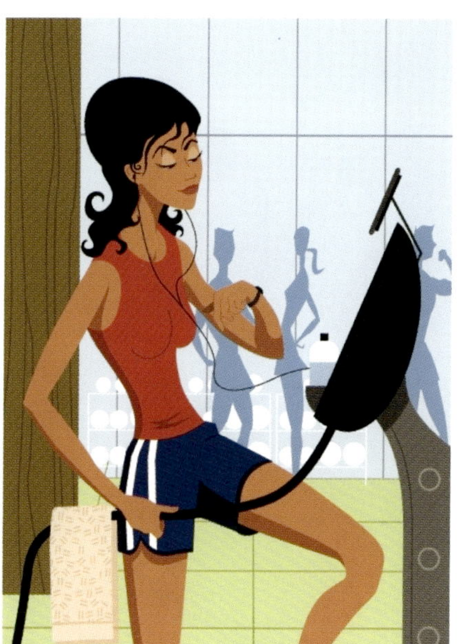

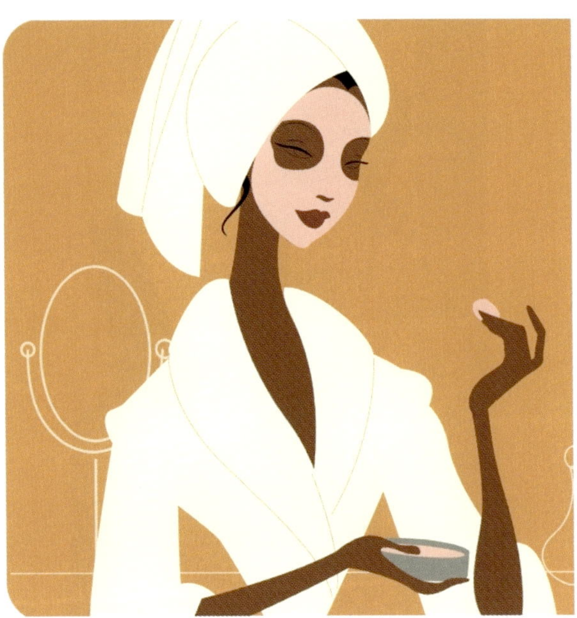

Not Just a Pretty Base...

Everyone knows someone who wears the wrong colour foundation and lives with an eternal tidemark around their jaw line. The mistake most women make is in thinking that foundation is to give colour.

Well, the big news is that it ain't.

Foundation should match your own skin tone to smooth over tiny imperfections and give a more even canvas for your make-up. A darker-than-you-need foundation won't help you look tanned and healthy, it'll make you look downright weird. Look out for 'treatment' foundations that protect and nourish your skin, and newer still idiot-proof foundations that will adjust their colour to your skin tone.

Ten Steps to Skin Heaven

1. Apply a light moisturiser on your face before you even think about applying your foundation. Without something to help it glide, you'll be scrubbing it in till dawn.

2. Put a twenty-pence-piece sized amount into the palm of your clean hand. If your hands aren't clean, your fingers' history goes straight onto your face; think putting out the rubbish, weeding the flower-bed, picking that… oh, never mind.

3. Add a same-sized amount of glow lotion to the foundation in your hand.

4. Mix the two together using your sparkly clean fingers until they are blended completely.

5. Apply in dabs to your face without rubbing.

6. As soon as the foundation is on your face, stroke it into your skin with your fingers as you would a moisturiser in upward motions. Spend time doing this.

7. Ensure the foundation mix is smoothed right up to your hairline on your forehead and right down to just below the jawline.

8. Treat the skin under your eyes like crêpe paper – go gently, gently and even more gently.

9. Use as much daylight as is available to check for unevenness, and if you find it, blend it out.

10. Do not, under any circumstance, be tempted to 'seal' it with powder. We're aiming for luminous here, not set solid.

Sherlock Won't Spot Your Disguise

Under-eye bags larger than suitcases? Zits making a bid for face domination? The downside to these tricky little problems is that there are no truly instant cures. The upside? Cunning disguise is your best friend…

Help! I Can't See My Cheeks…

• Look no further than your fridge for a cold but quick way to reduce puffiness around the eyes. A couple of ice cubes wrapped in a hanky pressed against those baggies will have them screaming for mercy.

• Eye masks that are made specifically to tame the downward journey of your under-eye area should be kept in the fridge for emergency use.

• A creamy concealer will cover up any dark circles. Look out for the words 'light reflective' on the packaging, as they contain reflecting particles that bounce away darkness.

• Best buys for concealers are liquid with a brush at the end for precision cover-ups.

• A soft-as-butter white eyeliner run around the inner rim of your eyes will give the illusion that you never, ever touched a drop to drink!

It's Life, Jim, But Not As We Know It…

- It's a bad idea to squeeze because the area becomes even harder to conceal, but if you must, make sure your hands are totally clean and dab the newly zapped area with antiseptic tea tree or calming, diluted lavender oil.

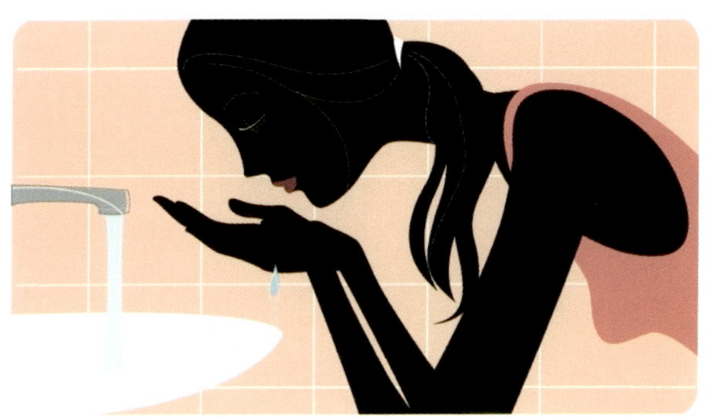

• Look out for a moisturiser specifically for combination skin. It is a myth that oily skin doesn't need moisture. What it doesn't need is more oil.

• Exfoliators can really come to your rescue by getting rid of dry, flaky areas around a healing spot.

• Careful with your cover-ups! You can't completely conceal a huge spot on your face, and smothering it with orange concealer will turn it into the Everest of zits. A touch of light liquid concealer is the most you can do.

• Glamorise your other assets, such as eyes and lips to draw unwanted attention away from your spot.

Underwear for Eyes

Is the skin under your eyes really so delicate? It sure is. It is 75 per cent thinner than the skin on the rest of your face, and has to put up with winking, blinking and weeping that strips away the few natural oils it has. The minute you realise this is the moment you stop dragging off your make-up, smearing away a mascara smudgie with licked fingers and scratching off tears with tissues at a sad film.

In the long term, the under-eye area is incredibly vulnerable to ageing, so what you do now will affect how you look in twenty years' time. Hard to hear, but best to know now while you can still save the day! So how do you keep future crinkles at bay?

Love Your Tender Touch…

• When removing make-up, dab the under-eye area with cotton wool to clean away residues. When removing mascara, shut your eyes and use gentle upward strokes with cotton wool and proper eye-make-up remover or Vaseline to gently get rid of the last traces.

• Avoid loading up the area with your regular moisturiser; it's a perfect recipe for claggy baggies that won't budge.

• Invest in a specialist under-eye gel or cream formulated to deal with delicate skin.

• Show your respect! Treat your under-eye area to an anti-ageing formula that will work with you to stay crease free.

• Don't bust your budget – thorough and light hydration is all that's needed.

Variations on a Theme

You want to go base-heavy because it's evening, and more must be better, right? Wrong. You want to slap it on because it has to last all day, right? Wrong. A really heavy look is never, ever good unless you are a) a model in for a photographic shoot, in which case you have your own make-up artist; b) you love the Morticia look; or c) – oops, there is no c).

Less is always more. A heavy make-up base intensifies any fine lines, makes your skin look unnatural and older and leaves you looking weirdly plastic. Using a sheer foundation mixed with a glow lotion will leave your skin able to breathe while giving it a sexy sheen.

In The Ring: Light v. Heavy…

Light: tinted moisturisers, ultra-sheer foundation, if:

- It's a summer's day.
- Your skin needs to breathe.
- You have great skin already.

Heavy: matt foundation, if:

- It's evening.
- It's winter and the light is low and dull.
- Your skin is uneven in colour.

Make-Up Artist Secret:

Apply a dab of moisturiser to
your base to help protect
and hydrate your skin.

Face Fact:

In the past, Chinese ladies
relied upon a jade face-roller
to keep blood circulation
moving and prevent
lines forming.

Top Beauty Tip:

Never apply a fake tan to your legs
directly after shaving. The colour seeps
into previously invisible hair pores, leaving
your legs dotted with brown spots.

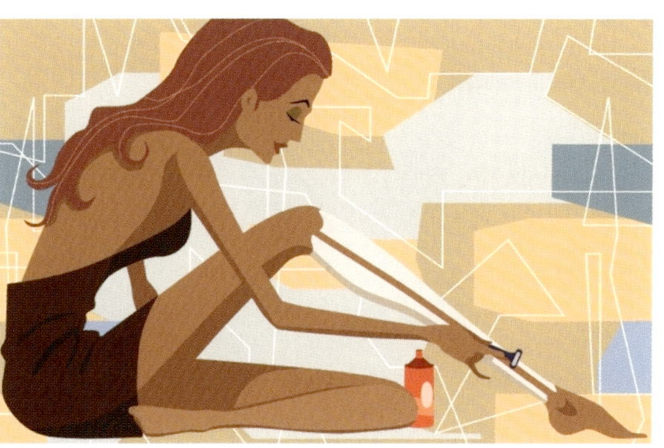

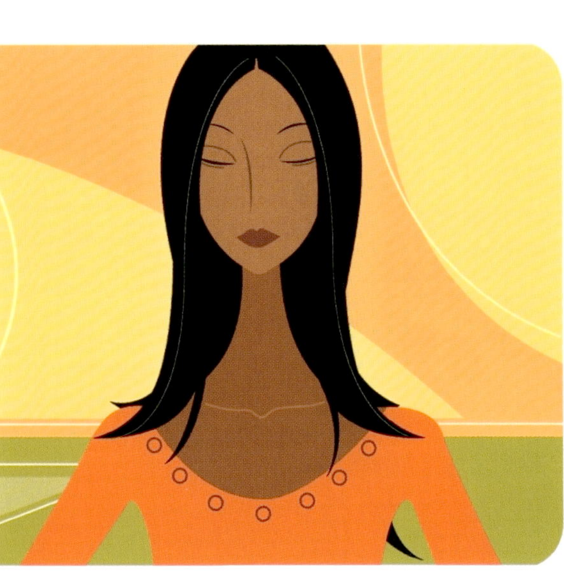

Jeepers Peepers!

Eyes are where the real fun with make-up starts! It's amazing how simple tricks with application can change your eyes from sweet 'n' sexy to downright dangerous! The old adage of choosing shades to suit your eye colour no longer applies because colours are more sophisticated and more adventurous application techniques mean that anything goes! Look out for eye-shadow trios – pre-packaged colours that will complement each other, taking the decision-making out of what goes with what. Watch out too for eye and cheek palettes that come with instructions on how to create a look – these take the guesswork out of making up and give you a professionally made-up look if you follow orders! From naturals and neutrals to high-octane acids, eyes can wear whatever takes your fancy…

Eye-Eye Captain

A few basic eye rules…

Small, Deep-Set Eyes

• The best trick in the book to widen and open up small eyes is to apply a pink, creamy eye shadow.

• Don't use a dark liner on the inner rim of the eye as it will make them seem even smaller.

• Curling mascara, or eyelash curlers, will help hold your lashes wide of your eyes, opening them up and giving the illusion of bigger soul windows.

Close-Together Eyes

• Use a light shadow over the entire eye area, such as a cream or beige, sweeping it up to the brow bone.

• Add a darker colour to the outer corners of the eyelid, blending carefully.

• Using an eye pencil, create an 'upsweep' line on the outer corners of your lids and blend well.

Big Eyes

• Eyes can almost never be too big, but using a dark liner on the inner lids will make them seem smaller.

• Don't go mad with mascara; choose a lighter colour, such as brown rather than dramarama black.

• Keep your eye colours neutral to draw attention away from the eye area.

Face Fact: Roman women cooked up a storm with their bear fat and lamp soot mascara… eeew.

Brow-do's

Bold and bushy can look blokey and brash. Thin and whispy is the reason why there are no electric tweezers and finally, the mono-brow: the ultimate in no-go areas for above-the-nose hair. Make-up artists will be the first to tell you that well-groomed brows are the key to beautiful eyes, and in a way they are right because they frame the whole area. Once you start grooming your brows properly, you'll never look back and won't consider leaving the house without your brow wax!

The Brow Beauty Rules

- Shape your brows with tweezers removing hairs from below the brows, never above.

- Softly, softly is the best approach – brows have a horrible habit of not growing back from an over-zealous pruning.

- Use an old toothbrush to brush your brows in an upward direction – you'll be amazed at what a difference this can make as it gives definition and shape.

• Invest in a brow wax to hold and maintain the brow line.

• You can use scissors to snip unruly hairs down to size.

• Pluck after a bath or shower when the pores are already open – it reduces the ouch factor by half.

Make-Up Artist Secret: For an emergency eyebrow touch up, sweep a small amount of mascara over them to hold them in place and add colour.

Get the Look

The Smoky Eye…

This is a fabulously sexy look for a smoulderingly romantic evening. Colours that work well for a smoky, seductive look are dark browns, frosty purples, deep greys and even black. When applying this look, don't chicken out at the last minute thinking it's all too over the top. It is meant to look heavy and is the only exception to the less is more rule. Just blend, blend and blend some more.

• Use a pale shimmery base, such as light pink, cream or ivory on the eye socket, blending well with a flat brush up to the brow bone.

• Blend a darker colour over the lid up into the crease area.

• Add a stroke of black kohl across the edge of the upper lashes and 'wing' upwards slightly at the outer edge of your eyes.

• Smudge the line with a cotton bud to look more smoky.

• With a thin brush, line under your lashes with the same dark colour, blending carefully.

• Line your inner rims with soft, black kohl.

Wear With It: A beautifully sheer, porcelain foundation with a touch of cream blush. Lips should be pouty, glossy and shimmering.

The Innocent But Dangerous Eye…

Also intensely seductive, the innocent look says, 'I'm not so…' but gives you masses of colour versatility. Try and choose colours from the same spectrum, i.e. greens and blues, pinks and browns, to help the blending process.

• Blend a neutral, soft colour such as cream, beige or palest pink over the eye socket and up towards the brow.

• With a slender brush, take a hint of metallic or iridescent colour, such as turquoise or green, and create a thin line as close to the lashes as you can possibly get it.

• Blend the line over with your brush until it 'melts' in with your base colour.

• Sweep the same iridescent colour under your lower lashes, again as near to the lash line as you can.

• Using dark brown mascara, lash it up so your eyes look huge and doe-like, and if you have a lash comb, rake it through to define each lash…

Wear With It: A sheer base mixed with glow lotion, pink cream blush to the apples of the cheeks and a baby pink gloss.

The Naked Eye…

There is an art to perfecting the neutral but gorgeous look, and mastering this will take you anywhere as it is totally adaptable by adding a splash more colour for evening. Start with three shades in light, medium and dark. Creams, light browns and golds work well.

• Using the lightest shade, blend across eye socket up to the brow bone.

• Taking the medium shade, brush it over the whole eye as far as the socket crease, blending really well.

• Using the darker colour, line around the eyes with the slenderest brush you have to enhance and widen.

• Use a modest amount of brown or black mascara on top and bottom lashes.

• Ensure your brows are in good condition for this look.

Wear With It: A tinted moisturiser with a brown or tawny cream blush to the cheeks, with a teeny smudge over the bridge of the nose. A cool, clear gloss looks fabulous.

Make-Up Artist Secrets:

Apply your mascara from the roots of the lashes to the tip using a rocking motion, then hold in a curled back position and count to ten.

Use a couple of tissues held under your eye while you apply shadows, especially shimmers, to stop your cheeks becoming accidentally sparkly too!

Face Fact:

Sweat and dirt from sheep's wool formed the **basis of** a face-whitening treatment in Ancient Greece.

Give your hair a holiday! Cut back on blow-drying which can dry out your hair, leaving it as dull as ditchwater. Halving your blow-drys will help your hair.

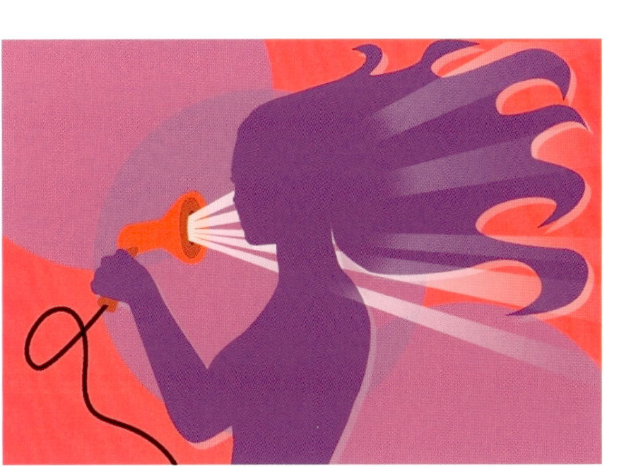

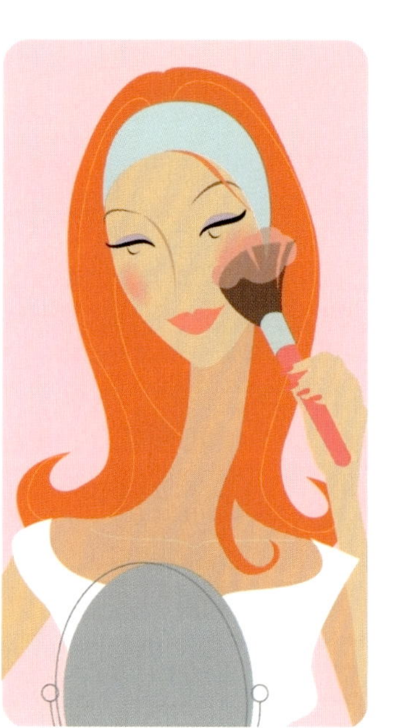

Hey, Cheeky!

B lush is the essential ingredient to lift your skin tone. Get it right, and a healthy radiance is yours. Get it wrong, and it's Aunt Sally meets a high blood pressure rush. Only the oiliest of skins can't cope with a cream blusher; if your skin is very oily, powder blush is your salvation, using a huge, soft brush to apply. Always focus on the centre of your cheeks when applying cheek colour – don't go way up high for Eighties-style cheekbones – aim for a soft glow to the apples of your cheeks.

• You want to look lustred, not flustered? Tone your blusher right down, and apply half of what you think you need. You can always add more, but scraping off is virtually impossible.

• Search for a cream blush; powder loves lines and seeps into tiny creases, making them seem bigger and more obvious.

• Try making up your eyes before your cheeks; it's easier to tell how much flush is needed.

• Liquid cheek stains can be tricky at first; they need quick application before they dry. Practise on your hand first.

• A neutral pinky/beige suits all, from deepest black skins to pale as paper; highly coloured blushers produce a dramatic effect that is generally inappropriate for a day in the office.

Make-Up Artist Secret:

Apply cheek stains and liquid blushers with a fat, soft brush for more natural and even-looking colour.

Face Fact:

Queen Elizabeth I used a white lead pigment called ceruse on her face and it was this that is believed to have caused her skin to pit and blister.

Top Beauty Tip:

Use a body oil in warm bath water to soften and intensively nourish your skin.

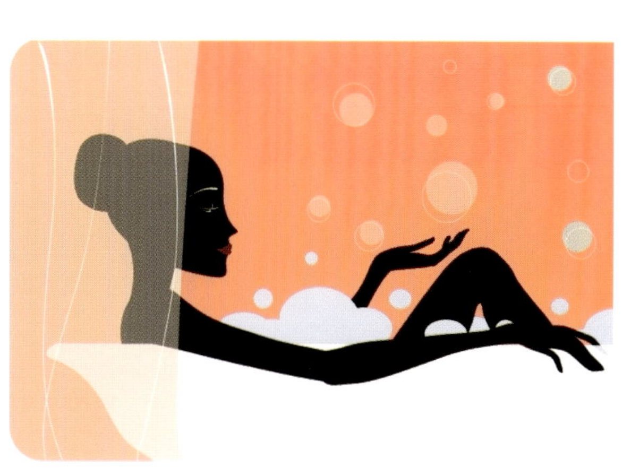

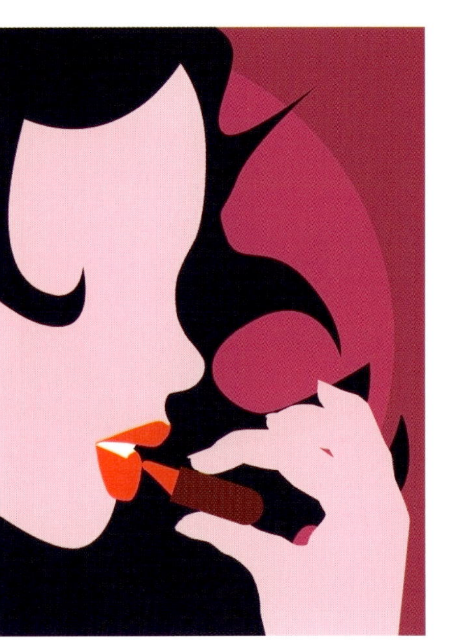

About That Pout!

There is nothing more sumptuous and kissable than a pair of smooth, plump lips. A really beautiful pout is an absolute showstopper. Here's how to get yours…

• When you exfoliate your face, don't forget to do your lips too; you can gently rub them with a flannel to get rid of dry flakes if you can't face the taste of your buffing lotion.

• Always protect your lips from weather extremes with a natural, mineral-free balm, such as beeswax.

• Drink lots and lots of water – this will plump up your lips and your skin.

- Matt lipsticks can be very drying – save these for special occasions.

- Sounds obvious, but pearly white teeth will always make your lips look special.

- Invest in a conditioning lipstick that will moisturise your lips as well as colouring them.

- So called 'lip-plumping' lipsticks have only limited success – if your lips are small and thin, you won't end up with a huge, juicy pout, just an oddly tingling mouth.

• A creamy lipstick can come in handy as an emergency cream blush; just apply a dot or two to the centre of your cheeks and blend.

• If you apply a strong colour to your eyes, don't even think about matching the same strength of colour to your lips – go gentle to complement rather than match, which can look over made-up and harsh.

• Change your colours according to season; a lightly tanned face can take a stronger shade than a pale but interesting winter complexion.

What to Wear?

Lipsticks and glosses come in every which colour. Finding one to suit you is purely a matter of trial and error, but when you find 'the one', buy ten if you can. Lipstick shades have a horrible habit of being discontinued just when you've discovered you really can't live without one…

Gloss

Gloss is easily the most forgiving lipwear; a nude or neutral shade suits everyone and gives a hint of sexiness while making your pout look soft and smooth. Be aware that we are talking sheer lip shine, not the so-wet-I-look-like-I'm-drooling Eighties gunge that went with shoulder pads and high hair.

• A pink gloss is the girliest of mouth make-up and it tends to suit everyone by adding a dash of radiance.

• Forget sparkling gloss: ridiculous, ridiculous, ridiculous! Who wants to look like they fell mouth first into the playgroup glitter tray?

• Accept that there isn't a way to make gloss stay –
be prepared to reapply often.

• Really sticky gloss rarely looks good – save the gloop
and go for a sheer gloss that doesn't make your mouth
look plastic.

• Invest in the new breed of keyring glosses that
mean you'll never be without the means to pout –
unless you lock yourself out.

Lipstick

Now we are all used to the gentler gleam of gloss, lipstick seems harder to get right than ever. Make use of testers at the make-up counters and stick to a few basic lippy rules:

• Oranges and reds can make your teeth take on a yellow tinge. Your teeth need to be ultra-white to carry these colours off well.

• Lipstick can 'bleed' into fine lines and cracks around your mouth making you look a bit drunk or damp. To stop this happening try a light layer of lipstick first, pat with a very fine powder and apply a stronger layer on top.

• You can use a lip liner to prevent bleeding by confining the lipstick to the lip area but it must be the same colour as your lipstick. Buy both from the same brand and ask for help at the counter with which liner goes with your chosen lipstick.

• Very dark lipsticks look beautiful with dark skins; if you are a pale face and you don't want to look dead, avoid them at all costs.

• Save time by being brazen. So your lippy leaves marks on glasses? So what? You need to reapply in the middle of dinner? Go ahead. Don't get obsessed – it's only lipstick.

Make-up Artist Secret:

Before you go to bed, slick a dash of Vaseline over your lips to wake up utterly kissable.

Face Fact:

Those inventive Roman ladies loved a dried crocodile dung face mask to lighten their skin.

Once a week, apply a conditioning
hair mask to keep your tresses
lush and healthy.

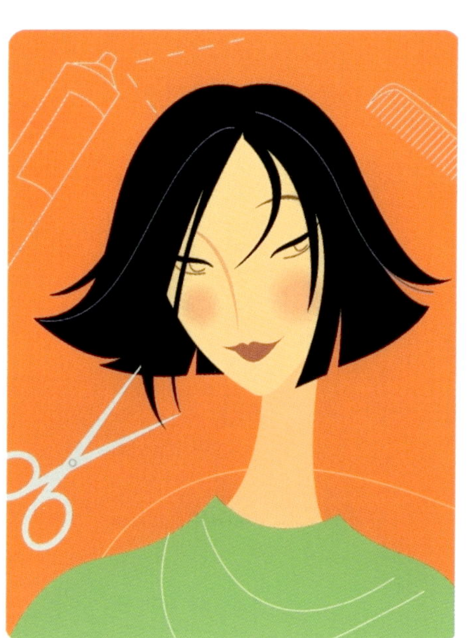

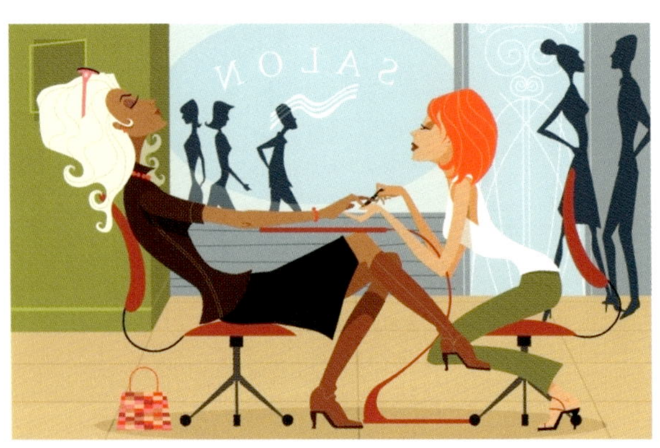

SALON

That's Nailed It!

These are the days of celebrity nail technicians, nail art, itty-bitty sticky things to add to your talons, nail conditioners, pierced nails, jewelled nails. Nails are shaped with odd names such as the squoval – a cross between square and oval. You name it, your nails can have it. But only if they are in tip-top condition and ready for action. Nail biters who are struggling to give up their nibbling addiction need to pay attention to the fact that, while your nails might make a light and crispy low cal snack, you're also chomping down everything you've ever touched that day. Like coins passed from who knows who to you via the till, like anybody's toilet-habit hands that touched the same escalator rail as you, or pushed the lift button, or shared a mug... get the picture? Not so tasty now.

Your Nail-Needs Kit

• An orange stick, to clear out unmentionables from under your nails.

• An emery board to file out shape and snags.

• A clear, conditioning or hardening treatment to wear under colour.

• A gentle nail polish remover.

• Nail-whitening tablets available from chemists for an ultra-clean look.

Everything else is an optional extra, including colours.

Nail Know-How

• Bitten nails are always best left au naturel; a slick of clear gloss is the most they can take.

• Regular filing will keep nails strong and less likely to break or snag.

• Always file in the same direction in a sweeping arc over the tips.

• When applying nail colour, factor in a ten-minute drying time between coats.

• Invest in a quick dry topcoat for quick finishes.

• Exfoliate and moisturise your hands regularly for super-smooth and hydrated skin.

• Invest in an everyday hand cream and always reapply after washing your hands.

• Wear protective gloves for washing up or heavy-duty work.

• For an ultra-conditioning night-time treat for nails, slather on hand cream and wear cotton gloves overnight.

• When filing, don't file down the sides of your nails as these act as a supporting wall to the rest of the nail.

Choosing a Nail Colour

Should nail colour match lipstick, shoes or even my coat? Will a one-coat really do the trick? So many questions, so little time.

There are no hard and fast rules to nail colours; wear what pleases you and if it matches your shoes, great. If not, what's the worry?

• An American manicure, as opposed to the outdated French manicure, will see you through any occasion. The difference between the two is that French has obvious over-bright, white tips, while American is a more natural creamy colour that looks like your own nail tips, but better.

• Metallic colours are difficult as hell to get off because the colour pigment tends to stain.

• One-coat colours should be for emergency use only – your manicure has more chance of lasting if it is applied in layers and finished with a topcoat to protect it from chipping.

• Pale colours are easier to correct if a little bit chips off as over-painting is less obvious.

• Neutral colours are a whole industry on their own, but steer well clear of beige nail varnish unless you want everyone to think you're attempting to break the world smoking record. It looks drab, faggy and frankly unwashed.

Make-up Artist Secret:

Whenever you moisturise your face or body, rub any excess cream into your cuticles for healthy, well-nourished nails.

Face Fact:

Medieval Italy reports
an ingenious beautician who
made ladies face powder
from arsenic. Husbands
who regularly kissed their
wives died!

Pretty feet never look grubby. Keep 'em
clean by soaking in warm water with
a little lemon juice.

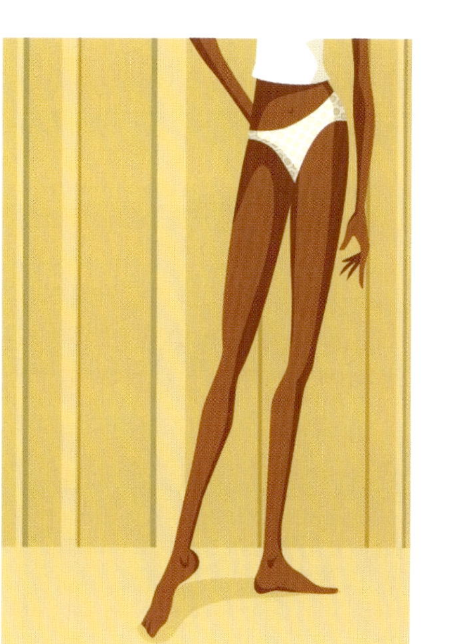

The best tip of all is to be happy with yourself.
It's what makes a true beauty.

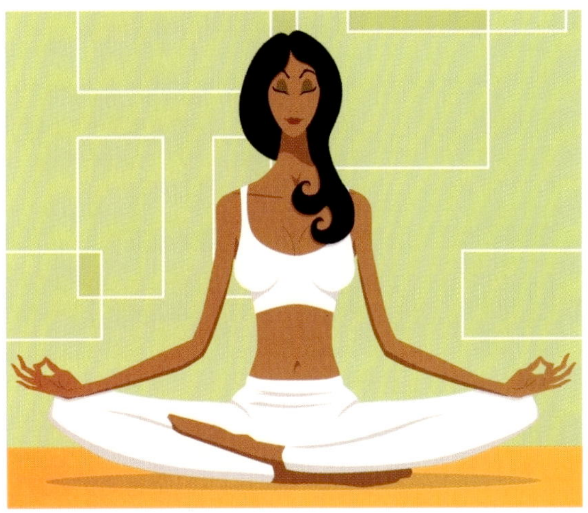